Build a Better Eater

The Picky Eater
Parent Survival Guide

Patty Canton

DEDICATION

To my sons, Ben and Zac, who inspired me to realize the importance of 'the food piece,' and to the many families I serve who share the same mission.

CONTENTS

ACKNOWLEDGMENTS

I would like to thank my family for their support and encouragement throughout my completion of this project. I am incredibly grateful for the many parents I have worked with who have shared their stories and experiences with me, and their beautiful children who help me rise to the challenge to keep doing and learning every day.

INTRODUCTION

Parents face many challenges, including feeding picky eaters. It can be frustrating to prepare a family meal that your child will not touch. You try your best to provide the best possible nutrition for your child, only to have him reject the healthy foods that you have prepared. If this sounds familiar, you are not alone! Picky eating is a common problem among children and unfortunately, it's a problem that seems to be getting worse.

Teaching our children to accept a variety of healthy foods is not necessarily made easier by our modern-day world. With an abundance of grocery store convenience meals and fast-food restaurants on every corner, children quite often develop a taste for processed foods at an early age, which contributes to their selectiveness when it comes to home cooked meals. What's more, children often become what is referred to as 'brand specific,' only eating foods from certain packages or restaurants. This can make feeding your family a very challenging task and can create a lot of stress in your home.

The saying goes that picky eaters are not born; they are made. Some parents note that their child has had feeding issues since birth. While I have heard this often in my practice, the truth is, if we practice any behavior long enough it becomes a habit. In the case of a picky eater, we're talking about an unhealthy habit.

After facing many struggles with my own children in terms of health and developmental delays, I came to realize the importance of what we put into our mouths every day. When I decided that eating habits were an important part of the overall wellness puzzle in our home, I was able to begin to make changes that have become a way of life for our family. This is not to say that our journey was easy…it was not. But it was worth it and is why I have made it my life's work to help others through the maze of picky eating.

To improve eating habits for kids we must first recognize that eating is a complex task, and to a large extent, a behavioral task. Knowing this helps us to be at a better place to manage the eating behaviors that led to the pickiness in the first place. While I will point out some of the complexities involved in eating, getting a good read on your child's typical behavioral response to feeding routines can give you a lot of information to determine what management approach may be the most successful.

This book is meant to be a guide to help you implement healthy eating changes while addressing eating behaviors for your child. It was designed to be a compact resource that you can return to whenever needed for helpful reminders and motivation to assist you with your picky eater.

While there is no one-size-fits-all approach to eliminating selective eating, there are some strategies that when used consistently can help to improve eating habits and eating behavior for children. Start where you and your child currently are in terms of accepting a variety of foods. Use the strategies in this book to help you refine your plan for tackling picky eating in your home. If you try a strategy and it doesn't work, try something else. The key is to keep on trying. It is my hope that you will find some of these ideas useful on your journey to building better eaters in your family.

Chapter 1

RECOGNIZING A PICKY EATER

Working with parents over three decades has taught me so many things, including to recognize that everyone is at a different place. When it comes to raising a picky eater, parents will differ a bit in their definition based upon their child's eating habits, as well as their own parental expectations for eating. Comparing your child's eating behavior to that of his peers might be what makes you realize that not every toddler eats a diet of only 5 different foods. Perhaps an extended family member has made a remark about your 'picky eater.' Or you simply recognized from early on that feeding your child has become a complicated matter that can end in tears, tantrums, and complete frustration.

So, what constitutes a picky eater? Every child is unique and will bring to the table (pun intended!) his or her own set of individual differences that contribute to eating habits and eating behavior. Still, you can typically spot a picky eater by some common characteristics:

Resistance/Avoidance

Children figure out at a very young age that if they exhibit certain behaviors, they can avoid the situation that they find to be unpleasant. If a child does not want to eat, he will find a way to let you know. If you don't give into his pleas, he will first escalate by any means necessary to get you to change your mind. Of course, this isn't always an issue with even tempered kiddos, but we are talking about picky eaters who were likely blessed with the strong-willed genes.

Picky eaters find reasons not to come to the dinner table and spend their time there either telling or showing you with their behavior how much they don't want to have what you have placed on their plate. They want the undesired food removed from their plate, and in some instances, removed totally from the table. The family dog knows to stay nearby during dinner as mealtime remnants are often cast his way by the little one. I have worked with children who even become upset when their parent is eating a salad next to them, and they will not calm down until the salad is moved. Many kids have also mastered the art of stalling to avoid eating unwanted foods. They may try to distract their parents with conversation, and more likely with their behavior. When behavior escalates at mealtime, it is no longer about the food, but instead about managing the behavior.

Self-limiting to certain food groups/textures

Selective feeders often eat from the 'white foods' group, wanting only chicken nuggets, fries, breads, waffles…you get the idea here. They cringe at the mention of vegetables and see anything with a vibrant color on their plate as an invader. They gravitate to carbohydrates, and steer clear of anything that looks remotely healthy.

Food pickiness often includes preferring certain food textures over others, whether it be crunchy foods or eating only pureed foods. Eating out can be a challenge, as the picky eater will only eat his burger or pizza from certain restaurants. Having food prepared 'incorrectly' can lead to meltdowns, making for a less than pleasant family dining experience.

Too often, parents find themselves performing as 'short order cooks,' sometimes preparing the child's favorite (and only eaten) foods, as well as making a separate dinner for mom and dad. It can be easy to get into a pattern of doing this to ensure that the picky eater does eat, as well as to avoid potential meltdowns. Before we know it, one day turns into the next, months go by, and a few years later our picky eater is still eating the same 5 or so foods while we are preparing a separate meal for the non-picky crew. While this situation occurs in more extreme instances of picky eating, I have seen these children often in my practice. I vividly remember a mother telling me that she prepared three different meals each night to accommodate all the members of the family. Sounds exhausting! The good news is that simplifying and lessening food preparation is another positive outcome when addressing picky eating.

Picky eaters often tend to experience what we refer to as 'food jags,' getting stuck on eating less than a handful of foods for short periods of time. It can be upsetting for parents whose child is already on the low end of the growth chart when the child further limits his diet. Well-intentioned family members and even the pediatrician can further complicate matters by suggesting that the picky eater be allowed to eat whatever he chooses to take in enough calories. Years ago, the first pediatrician for my sons suggested that because they were small for their ages, I should "let them eat hot dogs every day if that's what they wanted." This is the exact opposite of what helps a child learn to branch out in his diet to get the nutrients that he needs for a healthy mind and body.

Temperamental Extremes

There seem to be some similarities in the personalities of picky eaters. High intensity, or what I commonly refer to as 'big feeling' kids are often those who tend to be more limited in their diets and more vocal and resistant to accepting or trying foods out of their comfort zone. Many of these intense responders also have a short fuse, in that it doesn't take a lot for them to express their feelings. Frankly, if your child's strong temperament shows itself in other settings, you will likely see big responses from him when it comes to picky eating and feeding routines.

Children who are slower to adapt to changes by nature also tend to have feeding difficulties. Seeing new foods on their plate and even new brands of foods can take some time getting used to and often these changes are met with a high level of resistance. Incidentally, as parents we often adapt to our child's personality somewhat to comfort and appease them, but when it comes to routines including feeding, this can set us up for further difficulties. Don't get me wrong…a strong-willed nature and a resistance to try new things, matched with an uncanny sense of knowing just how to push parent buttons, can make feeding these kiddos a monumental task.

Sensory Sensitivity

The role of a child's sensory system is important, yet often overlooked when it comes to addressing overly particular eating. I've already mentioned that eating is a complex behavioral task, but it is also a complex sensory task. The task of eating requires the use of all our senses. Sometimes the sensory overload with how the food looks, along with how it smells, can impact a child's willingness to eat even before the food reaches their taste buds. Many children prefer only certain textures and flavors, and some have issues with the temperature of their food.

Sensory defensiveness often goes undiscovered unless evaluated by an occupational therapist or similar allied health professional. The truth is, addressing sensory issues can not only help parents to better understand their child's feeding and other daily living skills, it can help a child to regulate his responses toward more appropriate levels.

Here are some behaviors that may indicate a possible sensory processing difficulty as related to feeding for your child. While this list is not comprehensive, if any of these items raise a red flag for you about your child, it may warrant further investigation.

Your Child May:

1. Cover his ears with loud noises or noises that do not seem to bother others in the environment

2. Get easily upset by others at the table with chewing, silverware clanging against dishes, volume of voices or background noise (e.g., music or television)

3. Cover or close his eyes with too much visual stimulation and sensory overload

4. Have difficulty tolerating wet, sticky, or messy face or hands

5. Hold his nose, gag, or vomit with presented foods

Sensory issues vary among individuals, and often show up in different spheres for a child including home, school, and social interactions.

If you have sensory concerns for your child, talk with his doctor or another qualified professional to seek out appropriate support and resources.

Chapter 2

WHY IS MY CHILD PICKY?

Like Mother, Like Daughter…Like Father, Like Son

Even if we can't prove that genetics contribute to being picky, we do know that temperament or personality is inherited. If you are a parent with 'big feelings', then you are likely to have a child with 'big feelings.' If you have a 'big feelings' child who always lets you know where he stands, then you can expect for this temperament to show itself when it comes to feeding. This certainly doesn't mean that we can't alter our responses as we grow, it just means that we are more likely to respond a certain way and this factor should be considered in the picky eater equation.

An interesting point about genetics and taste is that our taste buds tend to be naturally more accepting of sweet and salty foods, with less of a preference for sour or bitter foods. I haven't met too many picky eaters who don't gravitate toward crunchy snacks and sweet treats. Still, it's important to keep in mind that our other senses of sight, smell, and touch (think texture of foods) play a large role in general food acceptance, influencing our perception of the actual taste of the foods that we eat.

Need for Sameness

You don't have to be an adult to be set in your ways. In fact, children develop a quick ability to settle into familiar routines. By the time a child is 2, he has developed a fairly comfortable routine, including what foods comprise his 'safe' regular daily diet. Getting comfortable in a routine can make it tricky to want to even try anything new. Moreover, that comfortable routine coupled with an inborn temperament often results in rigidity of routines and difficulties when the routine is broken. Let's face it, children need to feel that they have some control over their own environment (as do we all), and two of the biggest areas in which they can exercise control are going to the bathroom and, you guessed it, eating. While it is important to recognize and respect our individual preferences, there is no question that it is healthy for us to learn to be a bit flexible in our daily routines.

More about Sensory Defensiveness

We really can't underestimate the power of our senses when it comes to eating. We all have some foods that we love and other foods not so much. But even more so when we think of certain foods it can trigger feelings within us.

Picky eaters who also have heightened sensory problems tend to further limit their diets because of the way some foods look and smell. Add to that the texture of the food and even the temperature of the food and you have many factors involved in the process of eating. Children with special needs frequently show problems with eating related to sensory issues.

Food Allergy or Intolerance

Food allergies further restrict what a child can eat. Additionally, there are often food sensitivities or intolerances that may not show up on standard allergy tests but can still be problematic and contribute to self-limiting of foods for kids. Even young or non-verbal children know on some level when foods make them feel bad (or good) and so will refrain from eating them or even crave them to get that 'feel good' feeling. Interestingly, we often crave the very foods that are problematic for us.

We all have our favorite go-to or 'feel good' foods. There is scientific evidence showing that we can become 'addicted' to certain foods or more specifically the ingredients in them. This is something that is frequently noticed among children with special needs and is indicated as a factor that can increase negative symptoms for them.

Anxiety and/or Fear of Food

Believe it or not, trying new foods can be kind of scary for some kids. There is a condition known as Neophobia for those who have a very real fear of eating certain foods. I have not seen this once in over 3 decades of practice, but I frequently see children who have developed various levels of anxiety surrounding eating. This anxiety often shows up when there are expectations for a child to try new foods that he is wary of. Sometimes the nervousness associated with trying new foods results in the strong behavioral response often seen with some children.

Nutritional Concerns

Another common reason that can lead to feeding problems is nutritional deficiencies. Despite their parents' best efforts, many children do not get the proper nutrition they need because of the limited foods they eat. Deficiencies in certain nutrients can lead to an overall decreased appetite. Also, while the body doesn't know exactly what nutrients it may need, cravings for certain foods can develop as the body tries to get what it needs. Your child's doctor can help to identify any nutritional needs that may be contributing to presenting eating problems.

Mechanical Reasons

It is important to thoroughly assess children for chewing and swallowing difficulties. When oral-motor delays are present, children may be unable to properly suck, chew or swallow their food. Low muscle tone can result in weakness of the jaw, tongue, and lips, making it hard for children to drink properly from a cup or straw. Drinking or eating may be accompanied by excessive drooling. Speech difficulties are often a result of oral-motor delays. Strengthening oral-motor skills is an important part of treatment. A qualified occupational therapist or speech-language pathologist can evaluate and address any mechanical issues that may contribute to your child's feeding problems.

Medical Problems

Very young children and children with speech and language delays may be unable to communicate feelings of discomfort which can play a significant role in eating difficulties. The child may suffer from gastrointestinal issues, including reflux and constipation. Undetected problems in the gut including fungal or bacterial overgrowth can further contribute to appetite problems and feeding issues. Generally, when children do not feel well, they do not eat well. Talk with your doctor if you have these concerns for your child.

Learned Behaviors

Our children watch us and respond to us in certain ways. We set the initial expectations whether it be for manners, portions, or the issue here – what we want them to eat. They develop approaches to eating, we respond to that behavior and we either get desirable results, or we don't. When things don't go as planned, common parental responses may include ignoring, demanding, or bribing for feeding routines.

Sometimes, our efforts seem to be in vain and we end up with a picky eater on our hands. This is where behavioral strategies come in and why you are reading this book in the first place.

I always tell my clients these two things as we embark on a behavioral eating plan for the picky eater in question:

1. Every child is different and because of this, different kids respond to different feeding strategies.

2. I do not carry a magic wand (I wish I did!) and so cannot promise the implemented strategies will work. But there's a good chance they will.

Chapter 3

OVERCOMING CHALLENGING EATING BEHAVIOR

It's probably not going to be easy to transform your picky eater into a better eater. The problem likely didn't occur overnight, and it will take more than a quick fix to improve eating habits and eating behavior. Start where you are and take baby steps toward your goal. Experiencing small victories empowers you to keep going and making small changes toward your feeding goals means your child is more likely to go along with the program. With that said, let's get to work!

There are a few key principles when it comes to feeding children that when followed, will likely yield some positive results.

Set a Good Example

It is important that we recognize our own attitudes about food and eating in general. Our attitudes as parents affect how our children react. We can't expect our kids to eat a varied diet if we ourselves are selective eaters. I remember talking with a parent of a child I was working with whose goal it was for his son to eat healthier food, including fruits and vegetables. When I inquired as to the fruits and veggies currently eaten in the household, the father replied, "Oh, I hate vegetables." Children learn what they live, and despite what they may say, they really do look up to us. And, at least for a while, they follow our lead. We have to start with appropriate expectations for our little eaters, and we have to set a good example ourselves.

15

Manage Eating Behaviors

No one can argue that dealing with eating behaviors is typically not as serious as dealing with behaviors like aggression or other 'must manage right now' situations. However, it IS appropriate to look at managing eating behaviors as part of the daily routine. Addressing eating difficulties as behaviors is key to establishing better eating patterns. After all, who's in charge here? When mealtimes turn to power struggles, it is no longer about the food but instead about the behavior. How we respond in that moment is an important part of the feeding process. Plan for resistant behavior to occur, such as tantrums, refusal, and food throwing. Set appropriate expectations and limits for acceptable behavior at the table.

Case Example #1 Jeremy, age 4, eats a limited diet of mainly macaroni and cheese, chicken nuggets and yogurt. His parents have tried to introduce new foods, but efforts are always met with refusal and tantrums.

Strategy: Jeremy's parents will inform him of the new 'family rule' prior to mealtime. The rule will include that a tiny amount of a new food will be placed on Jeremy's plate along with his familiar foods. All family members will have the same 'new' food on their plate. Jeremy will leave the food on his plate without fussing or removing it. He does not need to try it at this point if he is just getting used to having it in his 'space.' Jeremy will be told that he will be removed from the table if he demonstrates negative behavior about the new food on his plate, and he will not have any other foods for the evening. Jeremy will be positively reinforced for complying with the new rule.

Structure – It's a Good Thing

Let's face it, most of us like routines. Having regular meal and snack times during the day will help your child to develop healthy eating habits. While there are some different viewpoints about grazing, generally allowing a child to raid the pantry throughout the day and eat whatever and whenever he wants means that he is more likely to be a picky eater.

Case Example #2 Emily, age 7, is famished when she comes home from school. She does not eat all of her packed lunch, and routinely eats her favorite afterschool snacks of chips, pretzels, or cookies. At dinnertime, her parents end up prodding her to eat certain amounts before she can leave the table. Requests are often met with whining and refusal.

Strategy: Emily's parents will provide a variety of healthy after school snacks. Complex carbohydrates like whole grain pretzels or crackers will be paired with proteins like nut butter or cheese. Portions will be monitored so that Emily maintains a healthy appetite for dinner. Parents will also let Emily know that she must eat an expected amount of food for dinner to have her evening snack of choice.

Being organized when it comes to what foods to serve is half the battle. A little preparation and planning can go a long way when it comes to snacks and mealtimes. Take time to plan meals and snacks before heading to the grocery store. Making simple, healthy menu plans and sticking to the grocery list both help to add to the structure for feeding. This helps to reduce our stress and increase the likelihood that our families will opt for healthier choices instead of foods void of nutrition.

Keep a well-stocked pantry, including readily available healthy snacks for mid-day munchies. Only have available what you want your children to choose from in the refrigerator and in the pantry. Remember, you choose what you are going to serve, and your children choose what they are going to eat, including the amount, from the foods that you prepare.

Little tummies fill up fast, so you want to be sure to fill them with healthy foods, including snacks during the day. So many little ones fill up on juice or milk just before or during mealtime. They are therefore not hungry at mealtime, and especially not interested in trying anything new on their plate. For older kids, it may be helpful to post a menu for the week (they can do some of the choosing).

Establishing Mealtime Rules

It's a good idea to establish some family rules around mealtime. Even if there are some rules your child is well aware of, it might be time to tweak them a bit if you are not getting the result you hope for with your picky eater.

An important thing to remember is that you choose what to serve, and your kids choose how much, what, and if they are eating from their plate. If your child refuses to eat and wants to leave the table, particularly if they are younger, you can teach them that they are able to make this choice, but there will be no food until later. In other words, they cannot refuse what's for dinner and then go to get another food of their choice within a certain time period after leaving the table.

Case Example #3 James, age 3, ate everything as a baby. When he was 2 years old, he began refusing previously accepted foods.He goes to the pantry immediately after dinner to request his preferred snacks. He is small for his age and his parents are concerned that he is not getting enough calories, so they let him eat whatever he selects.

Strategy: James' parents will offer James a new or previously eaten food 1 to 2 times a week along with familiar foods on his plate at mealtimes. They will structure eating routines so that James does not have a snack immediately after dinner, teaching him that he will have to wait until later if he did not eat a good dinner. If James is still hungry a couple of hours later, parents will offer 2 healthy snacks for him to choose from. James will be reminded at each dinnertime of this plan.

Try not to get upset or angry as children read our emotions and respond to them. Use family language of your choice to help your children establish good table time behavior. You can use words such as 'mealtime manners,' 'family food choices' or one of the favorite phrases I have heard over the years "take one bite to be polite."

We want to teach children to learn to take an appropriate amount of time and enjoy the eating experience. By the way, research shows that dinner is a pivotal time to introduce new foods to children with them being most likely to try something new at this family meal.

Chapter 4

STRATEGIES FOR BUILDING A BETTER EATER

Table Time Tips

When serving new foods, put just a little amount of the food on your child's plate. One-half to 1 teaspoon is a good rule of thumb to start with. Always be sure to pair the new food with a familiar, preferred food as you begin to incorporate these feeding changes. Sometimes presenting the new foods in the form of the child's preferred texture increases their willingness to try the new food. Be sensitive about providing slow transitions with introducing new foods and changing eating routines. We all want our kiddos to make improvements quickly, but slower, gradual changes or 'baby steps' help children to get comfortable with the new expectations, and this is more likely to lead to positive, lasting outcomes.

Teach Kids about Healthy Eating

There are so many teachable moments when it comes to raising healthy eaters. Sure, you can fly through the grocery aisles quicker sans your little ones but try to find those opportunities to engage them in the process. For instance, if you are in the produce aisle, have your child pick out a certain color fruit or vegetable that you can buy and prepare for dinner. So, if it's green beans, for example, everyone will have some of the green beans on their plate at dinner. Depending upon where you are with mealtime expectations at this point, you can either expect that your child leave the new food on his plate without throwing it on the floor, or you can have him touch, smell or taste the new food. Always praise your child for following the new feeding expectation. Teach kids that mealtime is for all members of the family.

Involve Them in the Process

There is no better way to increase the likelihood that your child will try a new food than if he played some role in the preparation. Even toddlers can add the grated carrots to the salad bowl or can stir the ingredients. Visit a fruit or vegetable farm. Let your child help you plant vegetables in containers or a garden. Have him help water and care for the growing plants, and even pick the harvest.

Along with actual foods, use other ways to help your child see these bright and beautiful color foods as a regular part of the daily routine. Picture books, toy foods, and games including apps are wonderful ways to bring 'the food piece' to the forefront for your child.

Make Food Fun!

I can't stress this one enough! The more we strive to change how we, and thus our children think about food, the more we can change their relationship with food and help them to value healthy choices for a healthy body. Use your creativity - presentation is so important to kids! Older children still appreciate a smiley face on their pancakes or their burger. Use small fruits and vegetables to make mealtime a little more fun while trying to get your child to try new things. And don't be discouraged if they don't try at first. It takes the average person a few weeks to develop a new habit, and this is a good rule to remember when incorporating new foods into your child's diet.

Develop a 'Tasting Plan'

When expecting children to try new foods, success can be improved by using a fun approach. I often ask children to tell me if the new food has a "small, medium or big" smell. Having children rate the smell of the new food helps them to better relate to the new food and seems to decrease food anxiety at the same time. Once we have labeled the size of the smell of the new food, I ask younger children to touch the new food.

We use a sticker chart or 'Tasting Tracker' to record all progress. For some kiddos, this may be for coming to the table or for leaving the new food on their plate. Again, start where your child is in terms of readiness when presenting new foods. The next step I take to help children get comfortable with a new food is to ask them to 'snake taste' the food. Even reluctant children are often very willing to try this quick touch of the tongue on the food after I have modeled the behavior for them, and I comment about how fast the snake taste can be! High praise and a sticker on the chart mark this huge step for very resistant eaters.

Making progress with these steps helps to reduce fear and build confidence in feeding for the child. When a child can comfortably 'snake taste' new foods several times throughout the week for a few weeks, then it is time to raise the expectation. I then request that the child take what I refer to as a 'mouse bite' of the presented new food. A mouse bite is just that, a very tiny amount of the new food. Always have a cup of water nearby and remind the child that he can take a drink after tasting the new food. Teach your child to focus on *"Bite, chew, swallow, drink water if you need to."* Choosing this self-talk over more negative "Eww, I'm not going to like this" type of language, helps them to work through the task more effectively.

Celebrate each 'mouse bite' victory just as you did with the 'snake tastes' and keep working at this expectation level until your child is comfortably taking mouse bites of new foods with minimal difficulty.

A very important note to mention here is that we want to be very careful when our children are learning to explore new foods that we do not focus on whether they liked the new food. Most children will typically say "No," particularly if vegetables are involved. At this sensitive place we want to only emphasize how great it is that they *tried* the new food. This is also a good time to remind your child that it sometimes takes our taste buds 10 to 20 times of trying the same food before we can truly decide if we like it or not. Again,remind them that you are celebrating that they tried it, that's all.

If you made it to this point – Congratulations…the legwork to support consistent progress has been done! You will know when it is time to request that your child begin taking 'people bites' of the requested food. You can also steadily increase your expectations for more of the non-preferred food on the plate to be eaten in combination with the preferred foods.

Overcoming Obstacles with the 'Tasting Plan'

There are a couple of places along the way in the feeding plan that I typically see picky eaters and their parents getting stuck. Keep in mind that the contributing factors to picky eating we discussed earlier will determine how slowly or quickly you and your child are able to master each level of tasting and trying new foods. Parents of extremely 'big feeling' kiddos often have to increase the structure to persuade the picky eater to go with the program. I had to do this with one of my children as he continued to eat very little at dinner, while holding out for his favorite before bedtime snack.

First, if your child is not eating well at dinner, you can let him know before the meal begins of the new family rule that he needs to eat dinner to have his evening snack. You may have this rule in place, but if you feel you are not making progress with your child eating better at dinner, take a look at the evening snack that your child chooses to eat. If it is carb heavy or a 'sweet treat,' restructure the evening snack, giving your child a choice of 2 healthy snacks that you present to him. If he refuses these, then he will be forfeiting his snack altogether. We need to teach our children that they need to eat healthy foods to have healthy bodies, and when they refuse a healthy dinner that was prepared, there needs to be some extra nutrition at snack time.

For some children, this will work well, and they may begin eating better at dinner. If things don't improve after a few weeks of this, you may need to play hard ball to see better progress at dinnertime. This was the case with my one son, who waited me out, and finally only responded to me wrapping his uneaten dinner and presenting it again at snack time. This was years ago but I still remember cutting and sectioning the amounts of chicken and green beans I wanted him to eat from his plate in order to have his favorite yogurt snack at the time. He eventually complied.

You may be asking yourself "I thought our kids were in charge of what and how much they eat from their plates?" Yes, you read that correctly. However, when we find that we are not making progress because our child will not budge, it is time to up the ante as a parent. Who's in charge here? You are, Mom and Dad. But again, no power struggles, state the family rules matter-of-factly, all the while presenting your child with choices (e.g., pick 1 of the 2 healthy snack choices) within the boundaries that you set.

Here's a quick recap of the specific strategies for transforming your picky eater:

1. Pair new with familiar – one new food at a time
2. Get children involved with food planning and preparation
3. Use a 'tasting plan' with your child
4. No forcing or bribing
5. Use a positive incentive/reward program
6. Everyone is involved…the same foods on all plates
7. Be creative and keep it fun!

Chapter 5

IMPROVING OUTCOMES FOR EATING

We've established some basic principles here to encourage your picky eater toward better eating habits. Of course, we know this will take some time and we can appreciate your child's individual personality in terms of how long it might take to see progress. Still, here are some additional things to keep in mind that can significantly increase your chances of improving your child's eating habits.

Make a Plan and Stick to It

Like anything else we learn, becoming a better eater takes practice. We as parents must be prepared for rebuttals and increased feeding behaviors as we implement feeding changes for our children. This can be very frustrating and make you want to throw in the towel but stay the course. Remaining confident and consistent with your plan will help you to reach your feeding goals.

Be cautious to avoid forcing or bribing your child. Many of us grew up knowing that if we ate our dinner, we would have dessert. I'm not saying this is a bad thing. But try to avoid using food as a reward. We just want to be sure that we do not place a higher value on sweet treats than we do on the healthy foods that nourish our brains and bodies. So, teach your child about 'healthy snacks' versus 'sometimes treats,' and encourage healthy snacks each day.

Many of us also grew up with the 'clean plate' rule. This one tends to be more problematic as we look to the current obesity rates for children and adults. Children innately know when they are full, so we want to be careful to honor this. Little kids tend to eat well for one meal or one day for that matter, and not the next.

These inconsistent behaviors are common for toddlers and preschoolers. If at any point you have concerns about your child's growth and development, consult your pediatrician.

Above all, be honest. That's not to say that you can't add some flax seed or spinach to your child's smoothie while they're not watching (go for it!), but at the same time we work to sneak in those nutrients, we want to provide many opportunities for our children to see foods in their natural state. An apple instead of apple pie, for example. Children need to trust us so if they ask what's in something, please tell them. Remain matter-of-fact when answering a question or two about the food but refrain from presenting a dissertation and don't allow it to turn into a debate.

Remember, it can take several attempts before your child even tries or decides they like a new food. Being patient, positive and persistent in your feeding goals will yield stronger results in the long run. Reward positive feeding behavior with praise, sticker charts, an extra bedtime book, 10 extra minutes on the computer, or whatever appropriate reinforcement works for your child. After all, the idea is to get them to repeat the positive behavior.

Managing eating behavior effectively by using structuring, consistency, and a bit of creativity along with a healthy dose of patience can go a long way to help parents with this important task. The habits you help your child develop will likely be with them for life so embrace this task as part of the 'well-being puzzle,' tackling one piece at a time.

Here are some quick *takeaway tips* to help with your family feeding journey. These helpful guides can be copied and kept handy as visual cues and regular reminders along the way.

10 Helpful Hints for Raising Healthy Eaters

1. Provide a balanced diet with a variety of delicious and nutritious foods.

2. Try to keep regular mealtimes, including snacks during the day.

3. Set a good example – eat a healthy diet yourself.

4. Avoid using food as a reward and encourage healthy snacks.

5. Organize your kitchen so that healthy snack choices are readily available to children.

6. Involve your children in shopping and cooking.

7. Plant foods in a garden or planter boxes with your children.

8. Avoid food additives – artificial colors and flavors, preservatives, excess sugar.

9. Watch for possible food allergies or intolerances.

10. Check with your health practitioner about nutritional supplementation.

12 Tips for Building Better Eating Behavior

1. Recognize our own attitudes about eating.

2. Manage eating behavior as an important part of the daily routine.

3. Be prepared and have a plan.

4. Encourage healthy eating while avoiding power struggles.

5. Establish consistent eating routines.

6. Define mealtime table rules.

7. Structure settings for success.

8. Use your creativity.

9. Teach kids about healthy eating.

10. Remain confident and consistent with your goals.

11. Reinforce appropriate eating behavior.

12. Be patient, positive and persistent.

Like anything else that we want to improve for our children, improving their eating habits takes work, commitment, and perseverance to yield lasting results. Best wishes on your journey. You can do this!

~ Patty

ABOUT THE AUTHOR

Patty Canton is a behavioral eating coach, speaker, and freelance writer, who never passes up the challenge to reform a picky eater. Patty has a background in child development, counseling, and holistic nutrition. She works with selective and adventurous eaters alike to help children develop a love for healthy food. When Patty isn't working, she can be found in her kitchen inventing new recipes. Patty lives with her family in the Central Ohio area. Visit her website at healthsmartconsult.com.

www.ingramcontent.com/pod-product-compliance
Lightning Source LLC
Chambersburg PA
CBHW061325250726
48657CB00003B/1053